Escaping My Killer

By

Mary Gorman

This is dedicated to the many doctors who saved my life.

I've opted to use just the initials of the people in this book.

A Usual Day

It was late October, at 4:30AM, I awoke
with my husband, it was a usual routine
work day; he got in the shower to get ready
for work, I did some stretching and warm up
before I got on my stationary exercise
bicycle, I rode that for fifteen minutes, then I
got on my stair stepper for ten minutes and a
cool down period. I had been doing this
routine for about a year, being that I was 37
and my metabolism had slowed down and I
didn't want to end up like my parents, who
both had health issues and were both
deceased before either was sixty-five. I
went to the kitchen and drank some water
then poured a cup of coffee for myself, by

then my husband had finished showering and was getting groomed and dressed, I went to the bedroom and picked out my clothes to wear and grabbed a fresh towel. My husband was dressed and ready to leave; he started work several hours before me. I kissed him goodbye and he left to go to work.

Alone in the House

Alone in the house, I locked the door, I went
to my computer to check my e-mail, I
logged into the computer and took a couple
sips of coffee. I felt a little upset stomach,
which was nothing weird I sometimes got an
upset stomach from coffee; I read my e-mail
and took a few more sips of coffee. Again I
felt the stomach upset. I thought, "Okay,
this is odd, I usually don't get upset stomach
this much over a few sips." I sat back in the
chair and I began to feel nauseated, thinking
to myself, "Whoa, what's going on with me?
The coffee couldn't have made me this
way." I started to have cold sweats, I got off
of the chair and I laid on the floor, I usually
laid on the floor if I felt I was going to be

sick or dizzy; I laid flat on my back and just laid still, I continued to have the cold sweats, I calmed myself physically and mentally, not knowing what was wrong, the best thing I could do was to remain calm. As I lay there not moving or thinking anything in particular, but just relaxing, the cold sweats subsided. At that time I figured it was okay to get up, I sat up at first and waited a minute to see if the nausea or sweats would come back, there was nothing, so I stood up, that was not a good idea, no sooner did I stand, I became very light-headed, the nausea returned and so did the cold sweats, I got back on the floor and laid back down; this time these symptoms were worse and coming on fast. I felt like I was going to vomit, I crawled to the closest bathroom, which was in the master bedroom, as I crawled, I kept thinking, "stay calm. What is wrong with me?" I got to the bathroom and knelt by the toilet holding my head in my hand ready for the purging to begin. It never did happen, at that moment I felt pain in my back, like someone took a board and wacked me in the back, it was very painful, I also felt like I wanted to have a bowel movement. I couldn't believe how I felt, all these things happening in my body all at once and how fast it came on. I laid down on the bathroom floor, the cold tile felt so good, I felt like I was on fire. I thought maybe this is a panic attack, I had those recently and they would come on at the weirdest times. But then the symptoms that was occurring right then, brought my thinking of what it could be to a halt, and all I could do was think to myself, "This isn't right, this doesn't feel like anything I've ever experienced." I decided I better call an ambulance. I crawled from the master bedroom bathroom to the living room where the phone was. I dialed the 911; the operator came on, "911, what is your emergency?' I responded, "I'm having chest pains, I'm nauseated, I feel awful!" the operator asked, "What is your address?" I told her, she said, "I am sending an ambulance right away." And although, I had no chest pains, for some reason, I felt I needed to say that. I hung up with the operator and crawled to the door and unlocked it. I crawled away from the door so I wouldn't block it. It seemed like forever as I lay face down on the living room floor, sweating and wanting to vomit but I had such pain in my back. I could hear the siren off in the distance, then it got closer and next thing I knew they were here. Not feeling any better by their presence, they took my blood pressure, which seemed normal, and they took my breathing, which seemed normal, I remained calm during this whole time, telling myself, "remain calm, don't panic, I'm safe, I will be okay." As the paramedics were putting wires with stickers on me, one paramedic asked, "How do you feel now?" I said, "I'm going to vomit! Get me something to puke in!" He grabbed a container that was sitting on the counter, the only thing that came up was the little bit of coffee I drank, the paramedic asked, "Do you feel any better?" I said no. They put me on a stretcher and took me to the ambulance, the other paramedics, closed and locked the front door. There was one paramedic who was checking my pulse and breathing, and my blood pressure as I was taken to the hospital.

In the ER

It seemed like only a minute I was at the hospital. The paramedics took me out of the ambulance and wheeled me into the emergency room, the nurses and paramedics put me on the emergency room bed, where the attending physician started asking me questions, while the nurses were taking my blood pressure, breathing and doing other things. The attending physician asked, how I felt right then, and asked me what happened that brought this on, He listened to my heart and helped me sit up as he listened to my lungs, he took notes and told me, "Just relax, I'll be right back." He touched my hand and gave me a confident smile and pulled the curtain around me. I lay there on the emergency room bed, trying to stay calm and at the same time trying to listen to what they were saying at the nurse's station. The attending physician came back with a nurse, "Mary, I'm going to have some blood work done on you, so we can find out what is causing you so much discomfort, okay?" I nodded. I asked, "Can you give me something for this nausea?" the physician replied, "Mary, I wish I could, but until we know what's going on, we don't want to make your condition any worse." I accepted that explanation and nodded. He left and the nurse asked if I needed anything? I shook my head, she put another blanket on me and pulled the curtain, I lay there with my thoughts thinking, "I don't feel too bad now." Then WHAM, like a ton of bricks I started sweating and feeling extremely nauseated and the pain in my back was almost unbearable. I started kicking my lower legs thinking maybe if I moved my legs it would help relieve this awful feeling, but it didn't. Then as soon as it came it passed. I just lay there in complete perplexity. "What in the hell is wrong with me?" Just then the Phlebotomist came in to take my blood, it seemed like she kept taking vile after vile after vile. I asked, "What will they be checking for?" She replied, "Well, the Doctor ordered a few tests so most likely, everything." I just looked away. The attending physician came back in, "Mary, another Doctor is coming by, he'll most likely ask you more questions. Just sit tight and he'll be here shortly." I nodded. While I lay there another round of sweats and pain and nausea happened. All I could think of was, "God help me." And like the other bout, it passed as well. A few minutes later, Dr. C showed up, he was an older gentleman, very well groomed, very well spoken. "Mary, I'm Dr. C" he said, "I understand you're having quite a morning." I nodded. Dr. C pulled up a chair and sat beside the bed I was lying in, "I need to ask you a few questions so we can better understand what is going on inside, okay?" I nodded. "This morning before you were brought in here can you tell me what you were doing?" I told him what I told the other

Doctor, Dr. C asked, "Did you take any medications?" I shook my head, no. "Did you do any drugs, like cocaine?" Shocked at that question at first, I shook my head, no. "How's your love life?" Surprised by this question, I told him it was good." He continued to ask, "Is there anything "life changing" going on in your life? Like a relative passing or losing a job?" I shook my head, no and told him, everything was the same. He got up and put his hand to his chin, he patted my shin and said, "I'm going to have one more set of blood work done." I nodded. He then went over to the nurse's station where I could see him, talking to a Phlebotomist; she immediately came over and took a couple of vials of blood. She smiled and took the vials and left. The curtain was open and I could see Dr. C looking over at me every so often, then he came back over to me, and listened to my heart.

It's a Positive

As he stood there, he watched my breathing,
while looking at his watch. Just then one of
the nurses at the nurse's station came over to
Dr. C and said, "We have a positive." Dr. C
then turned to me and said, "We know why
you feel this way and we're going to take
care of you." By then I was so sick and tired
of this coming and going of the nausea, pain
and cold sweats I just wanted it to go away.
One of the nurse's came to me, "Do you
want us to call someone for you?" I said,
"call my husband at 555-9999, tell him I'm
here and what's going on." The nurse said,
"I sure will, you just relax." Dr. C said
loudly to the emergency team, get the Cath

room ready, call Dr. K and Dr. H we got a
positive and this has to be done now.
The orderly's wheeled the ER bed down this
hall, to a dimly lit room, they placed me
where there was a woman at my head, She
said, "My name is Sara, I'm the Cath Lab
Technician, I'll be right here if you need
anything. There was a little television
monitor and some electronic equipment, it
was a comfortable calming room, Dr. C
came in, he was in surgical scrubs. He said
to me, "Mary, we have to use a balloon to
clear your vein, so we're going to go
through your big artery in your leg, you
won't feel a thing. We're going to numb the
skin so you won't feel where we're going in.
I nodded. Dr. K assisted him, I looked to my

right and saw a set of windows and a room, this is where Dr. H was, I think it was an observation room. The process began, I didn't feel anything until the balloon was passing by my stomach area, I got so nauseated. I told Sara, "I'm going to throw up." I started to turn on my side, in case anything came up, the Doctor's told me, " No, no, no, please lie still, we are so close to being done, I resumed my position of lying flat on my back and I remained as still as I could. I'm not sure if at that moment I died for a few seconds, but I remember, feeling no pain, no worries, no concerns I felt so at ease and content, I did see white all around me I felt like I was in a wheel chair or somehow being taken by an angel toward the bright white light, I could feel the softness of the angel wing against my cheek and I asked, "Is this what angel wings feel like?" Then that part ended. I opened my eyes and watched the little monitor, as I saw this little ball thing in my artery, then all of a sudden I could see blood rushing down into a vein on my heart. I thought, "Wow." That's all I could think. The Doctor's pulled the catheter out of my vein, and told me I did fantastic. Dr. C said, "You're going to the third floor where you can relax and recover, I will see you later, you just rest, okay? I nodded; I was so groggy from whatever they put in my intravenous.

In my recovery room, I was lying in the bed, going in and out of sleep, I opened my eyes and saw my husband there, I said, very groggy, "Hey, what are you doing here?" It looked like he'd been crying, but I wasn't sure, being how groggy I was. He said, "I got a call from the hospital that you were here." I said, "I'm okay now, you can go." He said, "I can stay." I said, "If you stay, I'm not going to be much company, I just want to sleep." He said, "Okay, if you want me to, I'll be back later." I nodded and drifted off to sleep.

I must have slept for hours, I awoke, but not thoroughly, still feeling heavily sedated, I looked over to my left I could see my husband standing not far from my bed, just watching me. Along with my Mother-in-law and Father-in-law, I said to my husband,

"Hey, what are you doing here?" He said, "I told you I'd be back." I asked, "What time is it?" He said, "It's eight o'clock at night."

"Wow, I slept the day away."

"Yep, you sure did."

"How do you feel?"

"I feel great! Except for this sleepy feeling."

Just then I could hear the loud speaker, "Visiting hours are now ending." A nurse peeked her head in, "Mr. Gorman, you can stay as long as you want. If you want, you can spend the night." My husband replied, "Thanks, I'll think about it." The nurse smiled an left. My Mother-in-Law and Father-in-Law both came to the side of my bed and said we just stopped by to make sure you weren't going to leave us. All I could do is smile. They said, "We're going to go now, we'll see you later." I just nodded. My husband asked, "Do you want me to stay." I shook my head no.

The next day, I felt a little more awake. The nurse came in with a bed pan, she said, "Mary, we noticed you haven't urinated since you got here, do you think you can go now?" I was surprised. I said, "Yes, of course." She helped me onto the bed pan and she said, you go ahead and go and I'll be right back to help you off. I nodded. I sat there, I didn't feel like I needed to go, but I figured I better try…still nothing. The nurse came back she asked, "Anything?" I shook my head, no. She asked, "Do you think you can make it to the toilet?" "I'll try." I responded. Then she saw all the tubes and wires that were attached to me, not to mention the "weight on a stick" they had on the place where they went in for the angioplasty.

She said, "I'm sorry, we'll have to give you a bag." I knew what that meant. It meant a catheter with a pee bag, uh! I hate those things. She left the room and came back with the "kit" in no time I was peeing in the bag, "Huh! I guess I did have to go." Dr. C came in to see me in the morning. "How are you feeling?" He asked. I replied, "I feel good, when can I go home?" He smiled, "Well, not for a few days. We want to make sure you're going to do well before you leave." I replied "Alright." I asked him, "When I was in the ER and the technician drew blood, what exactly were you looking for?"Dr. C replied, "Enzymes! When people have heart attacks they release enzymes into the blood, which tells us what is going on in the heart. Unfortunately, some people don't get here in time for us to check and they don't make it. Unlike you, who was smart enough to get here when you did." Dr. C checked my heart and breathing. "Okay, young lady, you rest and I'll be back tomorrow." He smiled and left. My husband then came in the room, "So how you feeling? Did the Doctor say when you can leave?" I replied, "I feel great, and the

Doctor did not say when I could leave.
How's everything at the house?" He replied,
"It's good." I asked, "Shouldn't you be at
work?" My husband replied, "Actually, they
said to take all the time I needed, so here I
am!" I smiled at him. We visited for a bit,
then he left.

Freedom

The nurse came in and asked if I would like the pee bag removed, "Yes, definitely!" Thus, I became pee bag free. What freedom! Still attached to the many tubes and wires, I wanted to get up and walk around but I couldn't because of the tubes and wires. The nurse came in and said, "Dr. C said you can become unattached to the wires, isn't that wonderful!" I agreed. The nurse pulled the stickers off of me as carefully and pain free as she could. All I had attached to me was the intravenous, and that I could wheel around with me. The nurse cleaned up the sticker mess and helped me to my feet, I felt like I couldn't catch my breath, she told me, " just take your time, slow calm breaths," finally, I was able to stand, feeling a little shaky, but standing. She asked, "Would you like to sit in the chair," I nodded, so she helped me to the chair. Then she took the mess and left. I thought to myself, "Wow that took some work." I decided, I think I'll try to look out the window; I got up and slowly, very slowly walked over to the window. Feeling exhausted, I slowly walked back over to the bed and got back in. "Wow, I am totally wiped out." How could someone, who had been exercising for over a year be so wiped out?" I couldn't believe how this incident was wiping me out. I lay in bed and watched some television. I realized I have to go to the bathroom, I looked over to the bathroom and thought, "It's way over there, and I have to walk it." I put my feet on the floor and took the trusty intravenous stand and I slowly walked over to the bathroom. I made it there, and took care of business; I then realized I had gotten my period. What a time for it to come. The heart unit of the hospital did not have any sanitary supplies on that particular floor, mainly because they don't normally get thirty-something woman in there who still get their periods. I told a nurse I got my period and asked if they could go to the maternity and get several pads for me; she seemed surprised, like I said, they don't normally get young woman in this unit. They did go get me a box of pads. That night I didn't sleep too well. I tossed and turned, I got up and looked outside, I watched some television, finally I got tired enough to sleep, I slept for a few hours.

The next day, I was put in a "regular" room, I had a roommate, the woman asked why I was in the hospital, I told her, "I had a heart attack." She replied, "My god, you're so young!" I said, "Yes, I know." She asked, "Do they know why this happened?" I said, "They said it was most likely genetics." "Oh my god." She gasps with air. For most of the day I was by myself, my roommate was out walking and talking with other patients, for some reason, I just didn't feel I needed to pry into other sick people's business, So I kept to myself. My husband came by to visit and it was getting close to Halloween, he asked me, "What kind of candy should I buy for the kids?" I asked, "What kids and why are you buying candy?" he said, "Because it's Halloween." "Oh ya! I totally forgot about that."

"Do you think you'll be out for Halloween?"

"No, I don't think so."

My husband stayed and watched some television with me; then my children showed up. They are all grown and they all came by at the same time. I was elated to see them. When they first walked into my room I guess they expected me to be hooked up to tubes and gadgets, and things sticking out of every part of me. But luckily I wasn't, I could tell be the look on their faces they were all scared. By the time they left they all looked relieved. My roommate was released sometime during the day and I wasn't aware of that. My husband lay down with me on the bed, I began to cry, I have no idea why I was crying. But I guess you experience some type of depression after a heart attack. My husband said, "It's okay, the worst is over." I guess I fell asleep and he left.

The fourth day, Dr. H was assigned to check on me, he came in and listened to my heart. He instructed me to get up and start walking around and move more. He asked me if I was sleeping okay. I said I wasn't sure, I think so. He said, "I'm going to prescribed something to help you sleep." I nodded. Dr. H left and said, "Okay, I'll see you tomorrow." I figured I'll practice, I'll walk to the doorway, I got out of bed and slowly walked to the doorway. It took me a moment to catch my breath; I turned around and walked back to the bed. Again, I had to catch my breath. My husband came to visit me, I told him the Doctor told me I should get up and walk around. My husband said, "Do you feel like walking?" I said, "Sure!" We left my room, and we walked a little ways out in the hallway, I could see the nurse's keeping an eye on me as I slowly walked. I found out some of the other patients on that floor had open heart surgery and that they too were walking around, but they were walking around a lot better than I was. "How could that be?" They had their chest cut open and yet they are walking like nothing happened. I didn't understand how someone whose chest was cut wide open, could walk around with ease, whereas, I only had an angioplasty I was finding it very difficult to catch my breath while walking. As we walked I would have to stop and catch my breath. We made it around the two main hallways then I told my husband, I needed to sit down. He helped me to the chair and I sat for a while. Then I got up and got in bed. He stayed and visited a while.

Halloween

We were quietly visiting, when I could hear
laughing and kids hollering out something.
We both went into the hallway, and all the
sick children from pediatrics came to the
heart unit trick or treating, most of them
seemed happy, they were given stickers and
stuffed animals instead of candy. It was a
sight to see, they were happy, but at the
same time I felt so sad for them, some of
these children were dressed in their
costumes but could only lie in their cribs
because they were so sick. Others were in
wheelchairs being wheeled around the unit.
Some looked so weak and pale, it looked
like they could hardly keep their heads up,

but if you looked in their eyes they were enjoying the trick or treat time.

My husband left for the night, I was tired from the walking around, so I got into bed and tried to sleep. A nurse came in and asked me, "Are you able to sleep?" I answered, "No, not really." "Okay, I'll get you something." She replied and she left my room. Minutes later she came back with a little yellow pill, she said it was to help me sleep, so I took it. I didn't think it helped me sleep.

The next day, they moved me to a private room. I asked the nurses if I could shower, they said, "No." I didn't really understand why, but if they said "No" I'm sure they had their reasons. I did bathe daily with a sponge baths, but I would've loved a shower. I asked if I could at least wash my hair, the nurse said, "Sure, that would be fine." Off I went to the bathroom sink. Oh! It felt so good to wash my hair, I went as far as putting a little make-up on. I came out of the bathroom and there stood Dr. H, "How are you doing? You must be feeling better?" "Yes!" I replied, "I feel so much better." "Good! Okay hop into bed, let me check your heart."

I did what he instructed me to do. "Very good!" He commented. "I can go home?" I asked. Dr. H smiled, "Let me consult with Dr. C and Dr. K and I'll let you know." "Alright." I was not thrilled with that answer but I guess it would have to do. About an hour later a new Doctor came in, she introduced herself and Dr. D. she wanted to find out from my point of view how I knew to get to the hospital, she was the one who informed me that I had a myocardial infarction (in other words a heart attack.) She asked me, "What was the one thing that you would say that prompted you to come to the hospital?" So I told her, "It was the fact that this, the symptoms, came on way too fast and didn't feel like anything I ever felt before." I asked her, "There something I don't understand, I was doing things in my life to prevent this type of thing from happening to me, I quit smoking over a year prior, I was eating right, and I was exercising 45 minutes a day, three days a week. How could this have happened?" Dr. D said, "There could be many factors, but we think it may have been hereditary." I couldn't deny that. She continued, "But you are very lucky you were doing the eating and exercising and that you quit smoking, it all contributed to a stronger heart, which is what saved you. If you hadn't done those things you may not have survived." She gave me a pat on the back and left. My husband came by with flowers, as we were visiting, a good friend of ours stopped by with flowers and more people stopped in. I really didn't question why everyone waited so long to stop by, I just thought they thought I should rest. After all the visiting and people coming and going, it was around

8PM. Dr. H came by, my husband was still there, Dr. H informed us that I could go home the next day, providing I did exactly as he instructs me to do. He said, "We are going to put you on a strict diet of no more than 20 grams of fat a day, and you have to take these pills, two for my heart and one for my cholesterol which he gave me prescriptions for, and he said, get daily exercise. I agreed to all conditions, I asked if I could return to work, he said, "Not yet." He also said, "No going back to work for a month." I said ok. He instructed me to see him after a month, and that he would be expecting me. I told him, "I will be there!" Happy to know I was going home, I slept very well that night.

Let's go Home

The next day, I ate breakfast and got cleaned up, I waited for the nurse to come in with the release papers, she did come in. I asked, "Can I call my husband to come get me?" she said, "Yes." I called him, he was there is a matter of minutes.

When I got home, my husband brought my suitcase in. I looked around, the house was in the same condition as when I was taken to the hospital a week earlier. My husband had shut down, he couldn't clean, cook or do for himself. I was shocked at first, but then I knew he had not someone close to him have a life threatening situation. I didn't complain, because I understood what was going on with him. He asked me if I needed anything, I told him no. I had always been one to keep the house tidy, not immaculate but tidy. I saw that it needed to be tidied up, so I started to pickup newspapers and put the pillows up on the sofa, my husband saw me doing this and he said, "You shouldn't be doing that, you should be resting."

"Oh for God's sake, it's just a few light items."

"No, now the doctor wants you to rest, and that's what you are going to do!" as he guided me to a chair. I sat for a while, my husband was busy preparing lunch for us. We ate lunch then he took the dishes and put them in the sink. Normally I would let this go, but the dishes were already piled up

from the week of nothing being done. So I
got up and went in the kitchen and started to
load the dishwasher, my husband just
watched close by. As I took my time
loading the dishwasher, I could feel a
pressure building in my chest. My husband
said, "That's it! You need to sit and stay put.
Don't worry about the dishes or anything."
I agreed, I could tell I definitely wasn't my
normal self. I sat and watched television
and would just get up to use the restroom.
That night I slept pretty good, the bed
wasn't hard like in the hospital.
The next morning my employer's human
resources person called me, she asked if I
felt well enough to come in and sign some
papers, I thought I was. My husband drove

me over to my work that afternoon, once inside, I sat waiting to be called in, the HR person called me in and I signed what needed to be signed. Then I thought, "I think I'll go say Hi to some of the people I worked with." I walked slowly to the few set of cubicles and quickly ran short of breath. I stopped for a moment then made it to the small set of stairs, I felt lightheaded and weak, I sat down on the stairs and caught my breath and decided I should just go home. I took my time walking back to the front door. My husband had the car right near to front door ready to pick me up. He asked, "Do you feel alright?" I replied, "No, not really." "I better get you home." He said in a worried tone. We got home and he helped me to the door and into the house, where he helped me to the sofa, and took my shoes of and gave me a blanket. That's when he told me I looked white as a sheet. By then I felt okay, but apparently I didn't look okay. I rested more.

Over the days I was at home, I would slowly do more things, still no heavy lifting or strenuous activities, needless to say this was difficult for me because I was a fairly active person. Not only did I gradually do more things, but I also had to change what I ate, choosing foods with a lot less fat content per serving.

Let's Eat

At first this was difficult, not to mention the food just didn't taste right, but I got used to it. I learned to eat the right things and use spices to give the food more taste and flair. My diet did not consist of just salads; I ate plenty of meat, lean meat. I went from whole milk to two percent milk. I love chips and salsa, my chips I changed to baked or fat free, and salsa has no fat, nor does beer. I started feeling back to normal. One of the conditions of being released from the hospital was to go to heart rehab, I agreed. At heart rehab, there were elderly people, of course young people such as myself were rare. The facilitator asked us to introduce ourselves and state what our heart issue was that caused us to have the heart attack. Some people stated high cholesterol, some stated their diabetes then it was my turn, I stated my name and was about to say genetics, when this wife of the patient shouted out, "I bet your reason was because you were doing drugs!" At first I got angry, how dare she assume I did drugs and that was the cause of my condition. I calmly said, "No, my condition was caused by heredity." And I calmly snubbed her. The facilitator said nothing, but the other folks in the room were thinking the same as I; that she was rude for doing that. She remained quite the rest of the time. I had to go to this class just once, but the rest of the rehab was exercise, where I was put on a portable heart monitor and was instructed to walk around an indoor track. I was allowed to use some of the other fitness equipment; I didn't dare thinking I didn't want to kill myself.

Four weeks of rehab; the Dr. determined I was healthy enough to go back to work. I returned to work and got back into the everyday routine until one night.

Not Again

I don't remember what night it was, but it was six months after my heart attack. I got into bed before my husband, then he got into bed. As we lay there just making idle talk, I got indigestion right below my sternum. Then the cold sweats and the urge to have a bowel movement. I told my husband, "Please call an ambulance, I think it's my heart again!" He called them, and they were there immediately. They took me to the hospital where I went when my first heart attack happened. At the hospital my husband told them of my heart attack and when it happened, they already had my records there. I could feel tightness in my chest, and my cold sweats continued; they

drew blood. My husband stood by the
gurney, I must have looked white as a sheet,
I could see the worry in his face. The ER
doctor didn't call Dr. C or Dr. H, this
concerned me, but while I was lying there, I
felt a release of something in my chest. Like
the blocked part became unblocked, all of
the feelings of tightness, the urge to have a
bowel movement and the sweating stopped.
I suddenly felt better; the nurse came by and
checked my blood pressure and breathing.
The ER Dr. came in and asked how I felt. I
told him I felt fine. The Dr. asked if I was
well enough to go home, I said yes. I was
allowed to go home. That left me confused,
if I were having the same symptoms and felt

the same way, why wasn't I treated the same.

I had a Suspicion

Before all this happened, I knew my parents were not the healthiest. My father died at age fifty-two from a massive heart attack, he was very tall and thin, he had hardly any body fat. My mother started becoming ill shortly after my father died, she was overweight and became diabetic which weakened her heart and she suffered several heart attacks. Paying attention in school helped me realize that I had a 50/50 chance of having heart issues, that was when I decided to change my eating and start exercising and quit smoking. But still as a teenager eating fast foods, not really paying attention to what I ate and the risk factors, I certainly didn't realize I was contributing to my own potential demise.

It's been over 15 years since those terrifying days. I have stuck to eating the way the doctors recommended, and yes I do go out once a month and have a "fat dinner," which can consist of cheesy, greasy, salty foods and yes, I do enjoy every bite of it. At the same time, you can feel the grease coat the inside of your mouth, which to me is gross. I have adapted to this life of less fat, I still have tried to exercise as vigorously as I used to but I find I still lose my breath, so I exercise not so vigorously, but I still move.

Gratitude

Every year at Halloween, I celebrate life, every day I am thankful to see the morning. More importantly, I am thankful to see my first grandchild being born.

When you come so close to dying, and feel what it's like to almost be on the other side, the calmness, the most wonderful feeling. You will never have that feeling here on earth, you almost want to go back, but doing so you will not return to this earth. When I experienced that moment, I was not afraid or scared. I felt wonderful.

I now realize that no matter how bad life's situations are and worries that don't really matter and material losses, those events and things are nothing compared to living and dying.